the
belly
book

a nine-month journal for you
and your growing belly

by Amy Krouse Rosenthal

potter style

introduction

What exactly is this Belly Book?

It's a sort of baby-to-be book, devoted 100% to pregnant mamas and all things belly.

It's part journal, part album, part keepsake—and all pre-partum.

You'll find places to document your cravings, gut feelings, and first kick. There are pages for preserving your ultrasound photos. And at the heart of it all: 40 slots for keeping a time-lapse photo log of your growing belly.

Sure, the idea is to fill this out as your belly fills out, but don't feel like you have to answer every single question and complete every single page. Even a sporadically filled out Belly Book will be a treasure for you (and your child) to look back on years from now.

—Amy Krouse Rosenthal

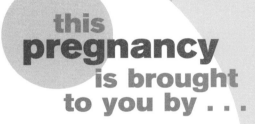

this
pregnancy
is brought
to you by . . .

name: _____

age: _____

this is my _____ pregnancy.

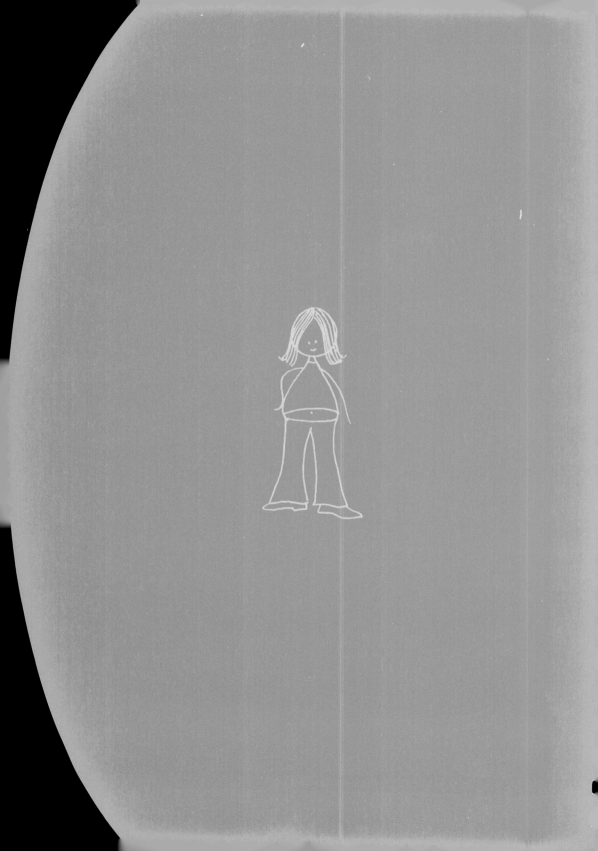

congratulations!

it's a . . . blue line!

Where and when I took the home pregnancy test: _____

_____

_____

_____

_____

_____

First reaction when I realized it was positive: _____

_____

_____

_____

_____

_____

How I told my hubby/partner: _____

_____

_____

_____

_____

Reaction: _____

_____

_____

Who we told right away and their reactions: _____

_____

_____

_____

_____

_____

_____

_____

This is our first baby. _____ Yes _____ No

How our kid(s) reacted: _____

_____

_____

_____

_____

_____

_____

When I plan to tell my friends/coworkers: _____

_____

_____

_____

_____

_____

_____

the first pre-natal visit

_____
(date)

My OB-GYN is: _____

_____

_____

Our due date: _____

My current weight: _____

My current belly measurement: _____

I'm thinking about delivering the baby:

___at the hospital   ___at home

___with a midwife   ___other

Here's why: _____

_____

_____

_____

Other notes from this first visit: _____

_____

_____

_____

_____

honey, can you please
come hold back my hair?

All the fun and gory details about morning (noon?) (night?) sickness: _____

_____

_____

_____

_____

Times of day when I feel the worst: _____

_____

_____

_____

_____

My stomach churns at the mere scent of: _____

_____

_____

_____

_____

Foods that generally calm my belly: _____

_____

_____

_____

_____

cravings & aversions

my first trimester chart

I've been seriously jonesin' for:

month 1

month 2

month 3

The thought of eating this is totally repulsive:

month 1

month 2

month 3

My philosophy when it comes to cravings:

_____mind over matter

_____give the belly what it wants

The weirdest food craving I've had so far is: _____

_____

_____

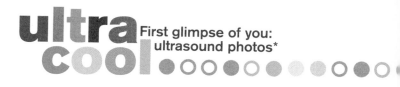

ultra cool

First glimpse of you: ultrasound photos*

photos here

First ultrasound date: _____

Pregnancy week: _____

Notes: _____

_____

_____

* Note: the ultrasound paper tends to fade with time, so you may want to consider making photocopies of the original for this page.

photos here

Ultrasound date: _____

Pregnancy week: _____

Notes: _____
_____
_____
_____

belly week 1

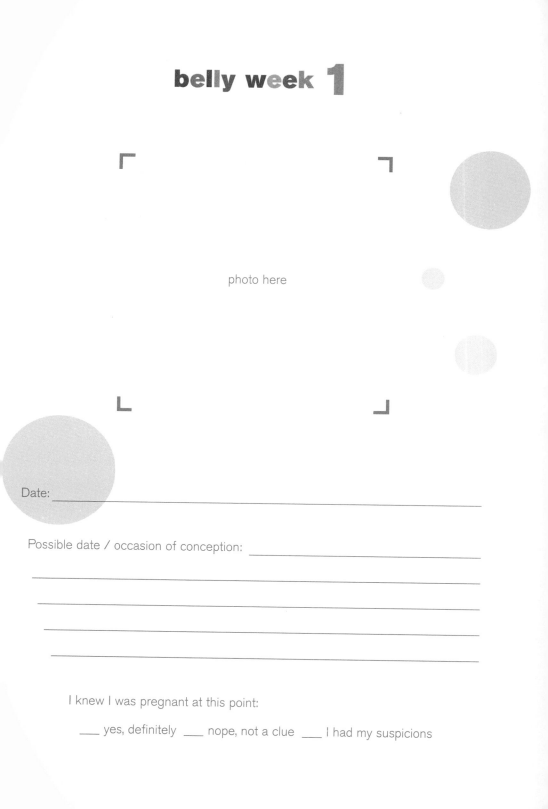

photo here

Date: _____

Possible date / occasion of conception: _____

_____

_____

_____

_____

I knew I was pregnant at this point:

___ yes, definitely ___ nope, not a clue ___ I had my suspicions

belly week 2

photo here

Date:_____

My earliest pregnancy symptoms (if any):_____
_____
_____
_____
_____
_____
_____
_____

belly week 3

photo here

Date: _____

Notes: _____

_____

_____

_____

_____

_____

_____

_____

_____

belly week 4

photo here

Date: _____

My current disposition:

____ sunshine and happiness

____ partly sunny, with chance of showers

____ hormonal hurricane

Other notes: _____

_____

_____

_____

belly week 5

photo here

Date: _____

Notes: _____

_____

_____

_____

_____

_____

_____

_____

belly week 6

┌   ┐

photo here

└   ┘

Date: _____

My energy level has been:

___ relatively normal   ___ a bit sluggish   ___ can't even complete a senten

Other notes: _____

_____

_____

_____

_____

_____

belly week 7

photo here

Date: _____

Notes: _____

_____

_____

_____

_____

_____

_____

_____

belly week 8

photo here

Date: _____

My complexion this week is:

_____ glowing   _____ green

Other welcome and/or not-so-welcome changes of late: _____

_____

_____

_____

_____

belly week 9

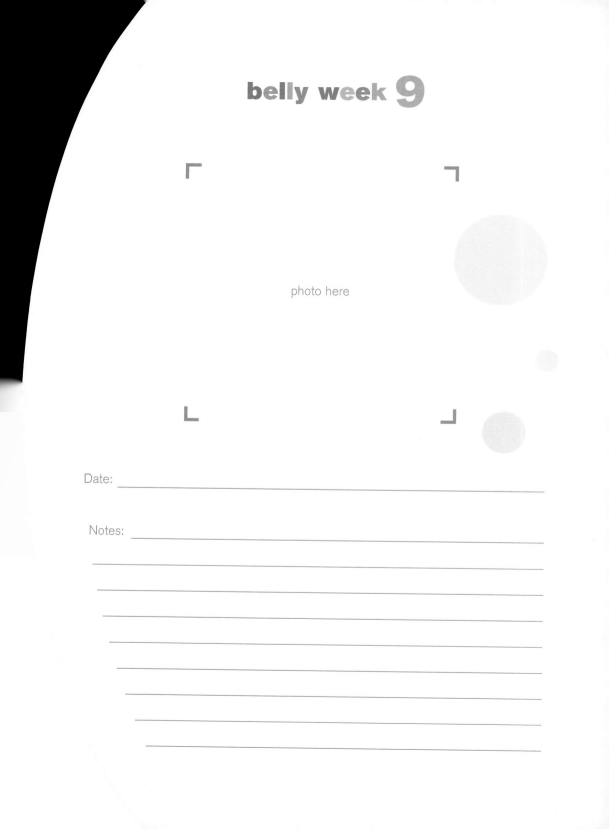

photo here

Date: _____

Notes: _____

_____

_____

_____

_____

_____

_____

_____

_____

belly week 10

photo here

Date: _____

My pants:

_____ still fit   _____ are slightly snug   _____ bring on the elastic

Other notable changes this week: _____

_____

_____

_____

_____

_____

belly week 11

photo here

Date: _____

snapshot of my life ○●○○●●○○○○●○○○○○

Music that I (we) have been listening to lately: _____

_____

Recent movie I've seen: _____

_____

Book I'm reading: _____

_____

Top news story at the moment: _____

_____

_____

belly week 12

[¬

photo here

L ⌐

Date: _____

this week marks the end of my first trimester

Reflections: _____
_____
_____
_____
_____
_____

Now we can tell everyone else: _____
_____

the stats

Appointment date: _____

Weight gained to date: _____

Belly measurement: _____

Estimated size of you: _____

Questions / Notes: _____

_____

_____

_____

_____

_____

_____

_____

_____

_____

_____

_____

Appointment date: _____

Weight gained to date: _____

Belly measurement: _____

Estimated size of you: _____

Questions / Notes: _____

_____

_____

_____

_____

_____

_____

_____

_____

_____

_____

_____

_____

Appointment date: _____

Weight gained to date: _____

Belly measurement: _____

Estimated size of you: _____

Questions / Notes: _____

_____

_____

_____

_____

_____

_____

_____

_____

_____

_____

_____

navel gazing

a few last thoughts about the first trimester

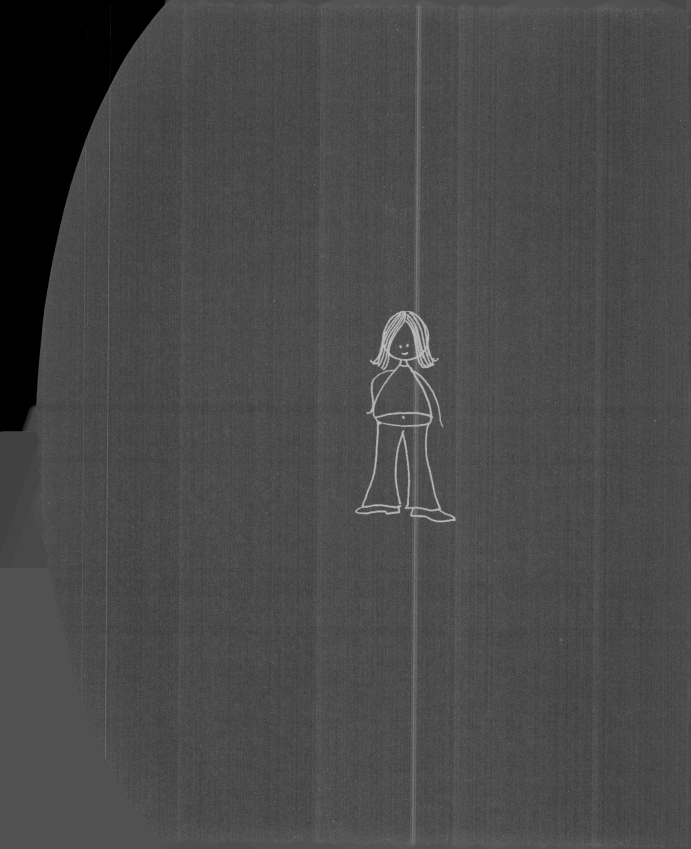

I 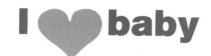 baby

Today is _____

It is a day I will never forget because we heard your heartbeat for the first time.

It sounded something like:

___ galloping horses   ___ a techno drum beat   ___ a miracle

Other thoughts: _____

_____

_____

_____

_____

_____

_____

_____

_____

_____

_____

_____

_____

_____

_____

au revoir, jeans

au revoir, any semblance of a waist

When I more or less popped: _____

_____

_____

If and when my bellybutton popped: _____

_____

_____

I'm starting to feel like:

_____ a fertility goddess   _____ Humpty Dumpty

More thoughts about getting big: _____

_____

_____

_____

My exercise regime: _____

_____

_____

_____

a few
clothes-ing
remarks

When I wore my very first maternity outfit: _____

_____

_____

_____

_____

My favorite maternity outfit is: _____

_____

_____

_____

_____

I borrowed maternity clothes from: _____

_____

_____

_____

_____

Record number of days in a row I wore the same heinous pair of stretch pants:

_____

_____

_____

boy or girl?
to know or not to know . . .

People say I am carrying:

___ high   ___ low

Everyone thinks you are:

___ a girl   ___ a boy   ___ twins

Personally, I think you are:

___ a girl   ___ a boy   ___ a boxer

My thoughts about finding out if you are a girl or boy before you are born: _____

_____

_____

_____

_____

_____

_____

My husband/partner

___ agrees with me   ___ disagrees with me

This is how we'll compromise: _____

_____

_____

_____

_____

I get a **kick**
out of you already

Week that I first felt you fluttering in my belly: _____

_____

_____

_____

_____

_____

A description of this new sensation: _____

_____

_____

_____

_____

_____

First time I felt you hiccup in my belly: _____

_____

_____

_____

_____

_____

_____

Week that you started to kick noticeably harder: _____

_____

_____

_____

_____

_____

_____

Times of day you move around most:_____

_____

_____

_____

_____

_____

_____

_____

I've noticed that these things seem to trigger you to kick or wiggle around: _____

_____

_____

_____

_____

_____

_____

second trimester
ultrasound

photos here

Ultrasound date: _____

Pregnancy week: _____

You are considerably more photogenic at this stage. I could clearly see the following
features: _____
_____
_____
_____
_____

The BIG question: You are a
___ girl ___ boy ___ stay tuned!

cravings & aversions

my second trimester chart

I've been seriously jonesin' for:

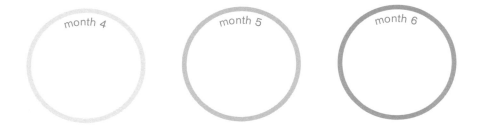

month 4

month 5

month 6

The thought of eating this is totally repulsive:

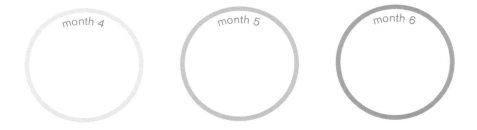

month 4

month 5

month 6

My current philosophy when it comes to cravings:

_____ mind over matter

_____ give the belly what it wants

The weirdest food craving I've had this trimester: _____

_____

_____

belly week 13

photo here

Date: _____

My mood swings are:

_____ tapering off, thank God

_____ totally justified considering how much my back is aching

_____ nonexistent—pregnancy has made me a Buddha (in size and spirit)

Other notes: _____

_____

_____

_____

belly week **14**

photo here

Date: _____

Notes: _____

_____

_____

_____

_____

_____

_____

_____

_____

belly week 15

[photo here]

Date: _____

Now that the hormones have really kicked in, my hair is:

_____ lustrous and full   _____ growing in some pretty strange places

More welcome and/or not-so-welcome changes of late: _____

_____

_____

_____

_____

_____

_____

belly week **16**

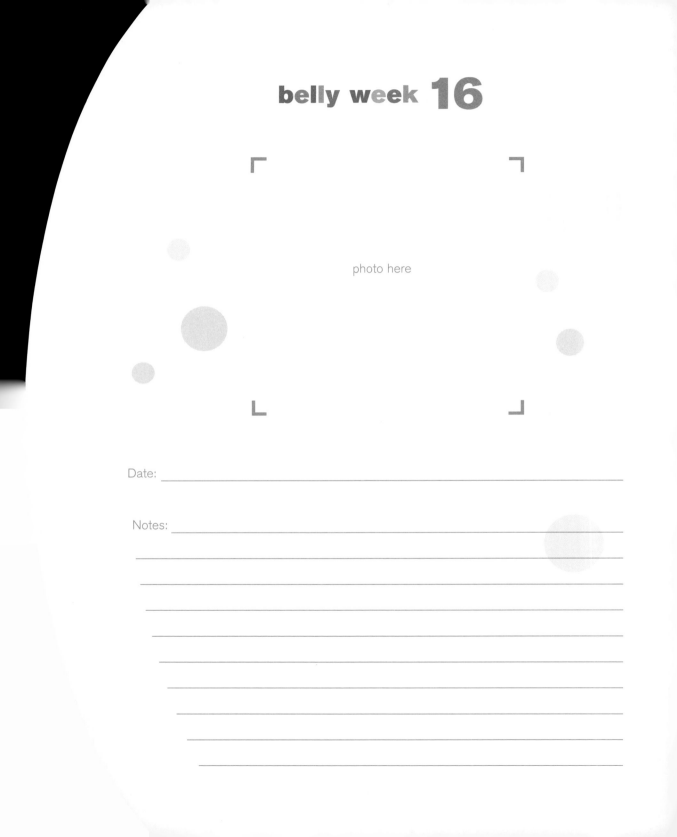

photo here

Date: _____

Notes: _____

_____

_____

_____

_____

_____

_____

_____

_____

belly week 17

photo here

Date: _____

My appetite is currently the size of:

_____ Rhode Island   _____ Texas   _____ the Louisiana Purchase

Other notes: _____
_____
_____
_____
_____
_____
_____

belly week 18

photo here

Date: _____

Notes: _____

_____

_____

_____

_____

_____

_____

_____

belly week 19

photo here

Date: _____

The thing(s) I miss most from life-before-the-belly:

____ wine with dinner   ____ a normal-sized bladder   ____ my ankles

Other notes: _____

_____

_____

_____

_____

_____

_____

belly week 20

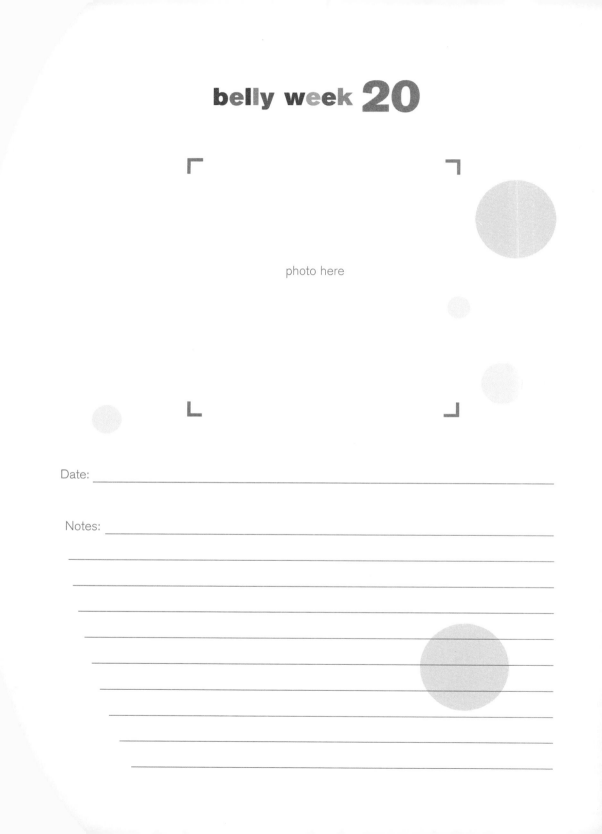

photo here

Date: _____

Notes: _____

_____

_____

_____

_____

_____

_____

_____

_____

belly week 21

photo here

Date: _____

I'm most comfortable sleeping:

___ on my back   ___ on my side   ___ Are you kidding? No way is comfortable.

I now get up to pee about _____ times a night.

Other notes: _____

_____

_____

_____

_____

belly week 22

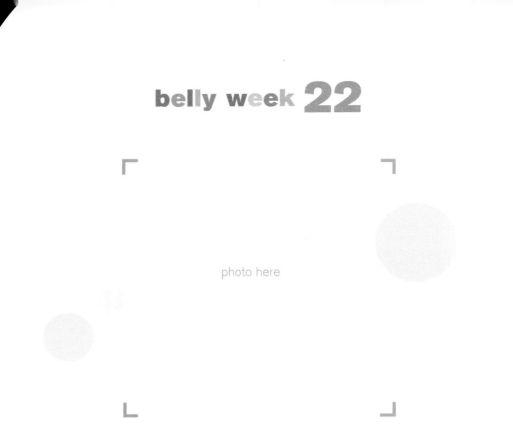

photo here

Date: _____

Notes: _____

_____

_____

_____

_____

_____

_____

_____

belly week 23

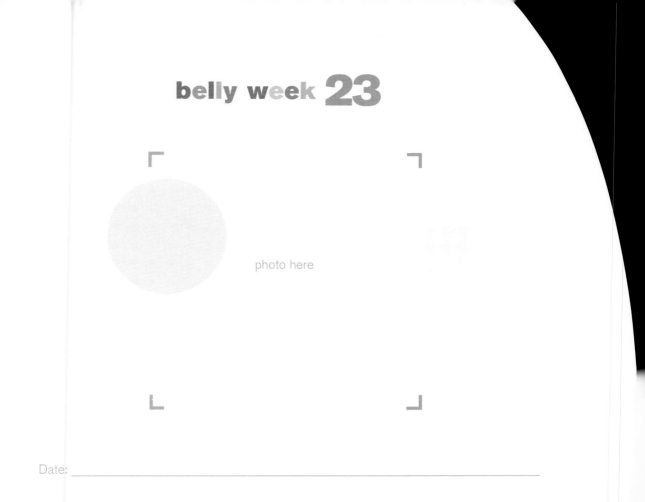

photo here

Date: _____

snapshot of my life ○●○○○●●●○○○ ○●●○○○○●○●○

Music that I (we) have been listening to lately: _____
_____

Recent movie I've seen: _____
_____

Book I'm reading right now: _____
_____

Top news story right now: _____
_____

belly week 24

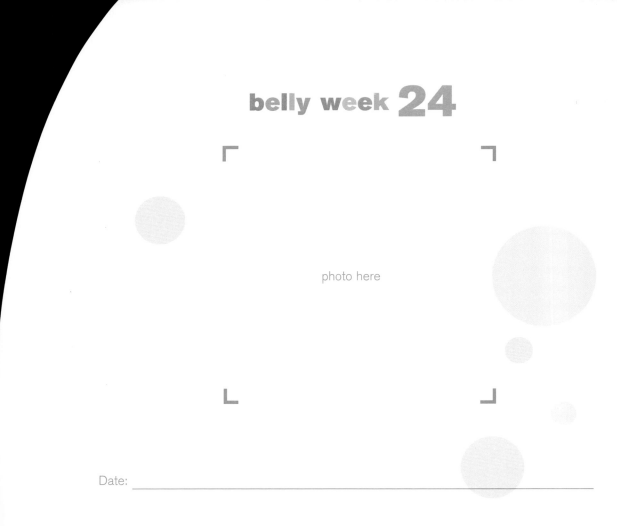

photo here

Date: _____

this week marks the end of my second trimester

Reflections: _____

_____

_____

_____

_____

_____

_____

the stats
the second trimester pre-natal visits

Appointment date: _____

Weight gained to date: _____

Belly measurement: _____

Estimated size of you: _____

Questions / Notes: _____

_____

_____

_____

_____

_____

_____

_____

_____

_____

_____

_____

_____

_____

_____

Appointment date: _____

Weight gained to date: _____

Belly measurement: _____

Estimated size of you: _____

Questions / Notes: _____

_____

_____

_____

_____

_____

_____

_____

_____

_____

_____

_____

pre-natal visits continued

Appointment date: _____

Weight gained to date: _____

Belly measurement: _____

Estimated size of you: _____

Questions / Notes: _____

_____
_____
_____
_____
_____
_____
_____
_____
_____
_____
_____
_____
_____

navel gazing

a few last thoughts about the second trimester

preg ed.

Type of childbirth class: _____

Instructor's name: _____

Number of classes I attended: _____

Who came with me: _____

_____ yes, I've been doing my Kegel exercises

_____ yes, I know that I'm supposed to be doing my Kegel exercises

Classmates I've befriended: _____

_____

_____

_____

_____

_____

_____

_____

_____

_____

my big fat
public pregnancy

People seem compelled to touch you.

___ don't mind   ___mind

First time a total stranger put his/her hand on my belly: _____

_____

_____

_____

_____

_____

_____

_____

First time someone gave up their seat for me and my big belly on the bus/subway (or performed some
other act of kindness): _____

_____

_____

_____

_____

_____

scooter, champ & mr. bubble

inexplicable belly/baby nicknames

Forgive us, but we've taken to calling you:

actual names
that we're considering for you

Boy names:

_____

_____

_____

_____

_____

_____

_____

_____

_____

_____

_____

Girl names:

_____

_____

_____

_____

_____

_____

_____

_____

_____

_____

_____

Other people's thoughts about your potential name: _____

_____

_____

_____

_____

the baby shower

photo here

You and I received:

	from	
_____	from	_____
_____	from	_____
_____	from	_____
_____	from	_____
_____	from	_____
_____	from	_____
_____	from	_____
_____	from	_____
_____	from	_____
_____	from	_____
_____	from	_____
_____	from	_____

a few momentos from the shower

cravings & aversions

my third trimester chart

I've been seriously jonesin' for:

month 7

month 8

month 9

The thought of eating this is totally repulsive:

month 7

month 8

month 9

My current philosophy when it comes to cravings:

_____ mind over matter

_____ give the belly what it wants

The weirdest food craving I've had this trimester: _____

_____

_____

you're quite the **mover** and **shaker**.

Times of day (and night) that you move around most: _____

_____

_____

_____

More things that seem to trigger your movement: _____

_____

_____

_____

_____

I've actually recognized your body parts moving and pushing against my belly (cool!): _____

_____

_____

_____

_____

When the term Braxton Hicks entered my vocabulary: _____

_____

_____

_____

_____

third trimester
ultrasound

photos here

Ultrasound date: _____

Pregnancy week: _____

Notes: _____
_____
_____
_____
_____
_____
_____
_____

the stats

the third trimester pre-natal visits ○ ● ○ ● ● ○

Appointment date: _____

Weight gained to date: _____

Belly measurement: _____

Estimated size of you: _____

Questions / Notes: _____

_____

_____

_____

_____

_____

_____

_____

_____

_____

_____

Appointment date: _____

Weight gained to date: _____

Belly measurement: _____

Estimated size of you: _____

Questions / Notes: _____

_____

_____

_____

_____

_____

_____

_____

_____

_____

_____

_____

_____

Appointment date: _____

Weight gained to date: _____

Belly measurement: _____

Estimated size of you: _____

Questions / Notes: _____

_____

_____

_____

_____

_____

_____

_____

_____

_____

_____

_____

Appointment date: _____

Weight gained to date: _____

Belly measurement: _____

Estimated size of you: _____

Questions / Notes: _____

_____

_____

_____

_____

_____

_____

_____

_____

_____

_____

_____

_____

Appointment date: _____

Weight gained to date: _____

Belly measurement: _____

Estimated size of you: _____

Questions / Notes: _____

_____

_____

_____

_____

_____

_____

_____

_____

_____

_____

_____

Appointment date: _____

Weight gained to date: _____

Belly measurement: _____

Estimated size of you: _____

Questions / Notes: _____

_____

_____

_____

_____

_____

_____

_____

_____

_____

_____

_____

_____

pre-natal visits continued ○ ● ● ● ●● ○○ ● ○ ● ● ●○○ ●○ ● ○

Appointment date: _____

Weight gained to date: _____

Belly measurement: _____

Estimated size of you: _____

Questions / Notes: _____

_____

_____

_____

_____

_____

_____

_____

_____

_____

_____

_____

_____

belly week 25

photo here

Date: _____

I feel compelled to talk about my pregnancy:

_____ anytime, with anyone who happens to be around

_____ only with other pregnant women or new mothers

_____ not much at all

Other notes:_____

_____

_____

_____

_____

belly week 26

photo here

Date: _____

Notes: _____

_____

_____

_____

_____

_____

_____

_____

_____

belly week 27

photo here

Date: _____

Right now my husband/partner is feeling a little:

____ overwhelmed   ____ overprotective   ____ left out   ____ ecstatic   ____ all of the above

Other notes: _____

_____

_____

_____

_____

_____

_____

belly week **28**

photo here

Date: _____

Notes: _____

_____

_____

_____

_____

_____

_____

_____

belly week 29

photo here

Date: _____

More thing(s) that I miss from life-before-the-belly:

_____ walking sans waddle   _____ my lap   _____ normal undies

Other notes: _____

_____

_____

_____

_____

_____

_____

belly week **30**

photo here

Date: _____

Notes: _____

_____

_____

_____

_____

_____

_____

_____

_____

belly week 31

photo here

Date:_____

I am now most comfortable sleeping:

___ on my back   ___ on my side   ___ I'll take it any way I can get it

I am now getting up to pee about _____ times a night.

Other notes: _____

_____

_____

_____

_____

belly week 32

photo here

Date: _____

Notes: _____

_____

_____

_____

_____

_____

_____

_____

_____

belly week 33

photo here

Date: _____

Notes: _____

_____

_____

One month to go! This is what I'm doing to prepare for your arrival: _____

_____

_____

_____ I think I'm officially nesting.

_____ What's nesting?

belly week 34

photo here

Date: _____

Notes: _____

_____

_____

_____

_____

_____

_____

_____

belly week 35

photo here

Date: _____

People say that my belly looks:

____ less pregnant that it actually is   ____ right on target   ____ like it's ready to pop

Other notes: _____
_____
_____
_____
_____
_____

belly week **36**

photo here

Date: _____

Notes: _____

_____

_____

_____

_____

_____

_____

_____

_____

belly week 37

photo here

Date: _____

snapshot of my life ○●○○○●●○○○○○●○●○○○○●○●○○○●●○

Music that I (we) have been listening to lately: _____

_____

Recent movie I've seen: _____

_____

Book I'm reading right now: _____

_____

Top news story right now: _____

_____

_____

belly week 38

photo here

Date: _____

Notes: _____

_____

_____

_____

_____

_____

_____

_____

_____

_____

belly week 39

photo here

Date: _____

Notes: _____

_____

_____

_____

_____

_____

_____

_____

_____

details of
your belly departure

My labor began:

_____ days before your due date

_____ days late (of all the nerve!)

_____ right on time

_____ none of the above (I was induced/had a scheduled c-section)

Where I was when the contractions started, and who helped me get ready:

_____

_____

_____

_____

_____

_____

Where I was when my water broke: _____

_____

_____

_____

_____

Total number of hours that I was in labor: _____

The Lamaze breathing class sure came in handy:

___ absolutely

___ very funny

So, this is what labor feels like: _____

_____

_____

_____

_____

_____

_____

_____

_____

_____

_____

_____

_____

_____

_____

_____

special delivery!

You were born:

_____ in a hospital   _____ at home

_____ in a birthing center   _____ other: _____

Epidural, au naturel, or c-section: _____

If I were to do it all over again, my approach would be: _____

_____

_____

_____

_____

_____

Who delivered you: _____

_____

_____

Who cut the umbilical cord: _____

Who was present during the birth: _____

_____

Nurses and helpers I don't want to forget: _____

_____

_____

How my husband/partner coped in the delivery room: _____

_____

_____

_____

Who came to visit us: _____

_____

_____

_____

_____

Other good stories and interesting details about your entry into the world: _____

_____

_____

_____

_____

_____

How I felt when I first saw you: _____

_____

_____

_____

_____

_____

_____

_____

_____

How it felt to hold you for the first time: _____

_____

_____

_____

_____

_____

_____

_____

_____

_____

_____

happy birthday!

photo here

_____
Your name

_____
Date and time of arrival

_____
Weight

_____
Length

your
footprints
here

belly epilogue

_____ I still look pregnant.

_____ Surprisingly, my belly is almost back to its normal size.

_____ I'm so happy you are here but I didn't realize how much
I'd miss having you in my belly, being so close.

Notes: _____

_____

_____

_____

_____

_____

_____

_____

_____

_____

_____

_____

_____

_____

_____

the end of the belly book
the beginning of you

photo here

All in the Family!

Your little one will love growing up with this collection of keepsakes by Amy Krouse Rosenthal.

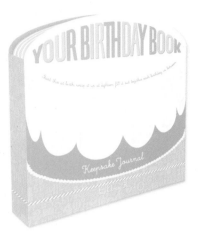

Your Birthday Book: A Keepsake Journal
ISBN 978-0-307-34230-0
$19.95 (Canada: $25.95)

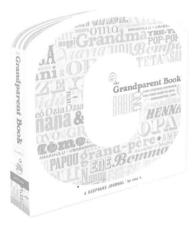

The Grandparent Book: A Keepsake Journal
ISBN 978-0-307-45310-5 (available on 8/25/09)
$16.99 (Canada: $21.99)

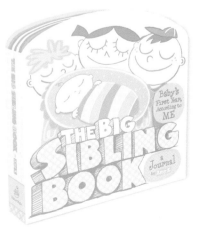

The Big Sibling Book: Baby's First Year According to Me
ISBN 978-0-307-46197-1 (available on 10/20/09)
$16.99 (Canada: $21.99)

Available at www.randomhouse.com, or wherever books are sold.